ISBN Paperback: 978-1-64873-414-4
eBOOK: 978-1-64873-415-1

Printed in the United States of America
Published by: Writer's Publishing House
Prescott, AZ 86301

Optimizing Brain Power

How Hearing Health Affects Cognition

Doug Dunker ACA, BC-HIS

Board Certified—Hearing Instrument Sciences

American Conference of Audioprosthology

Contents

Part 5

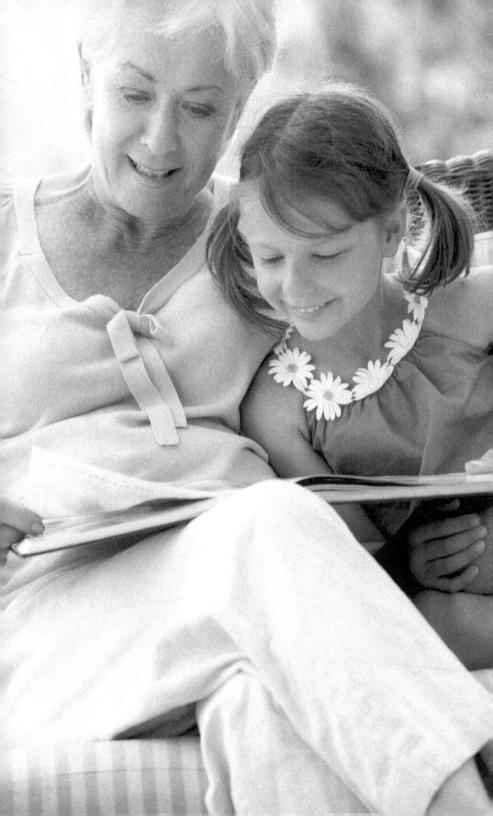

Preface

According to the American Speech-Language-Hearing Association, it is estimated that 48 million Americans have some degree of hearing loss or tinnitus. Yet approximately 36 million of them go without treatment.

- Are you concerned about the potential long-term effects of hearing loss?
- Do you want to keep your mind sharp and reduce the risk of dementia?
- Do you want to stay socially active and connected to friends and family?
- Are you concerned about how hearing problems can affect the overall quality of life?

If you or someone you know has responded *yes* to any of the questions above, please continue reading. The information inside these pages will help you understand how to live a happier, more active, and healthier lifestyle as you age.

Hearing is one of our major senses. In fact, it is considered the most complicated and intricate sense of the human body. Our sense of hearing helps us detect sounds in the environment, alert us to danger, and enjoy music and other auditory experiences. But the principal function of the ears is that they aid in the perception of speech, language, and sound-based communication.

Optimizing Brain Power demonstrates the severe implications of not treating hearing loss and explains the various treatment solutions available. The treatment for hearing loss also reduces the risk of dementia, depression, and falling while simultaneously promoting a healthier and more fulfilled lifestyle with increased physical activity as you age.

The Department of Health and Human Services has listed hearing loss as the third most common chronic health condition among seniors. Approximately one-half of adults between the ages of sixty and seventy and two-thirds of adults aged seventy to eighty are living with hearing loss. As longevity increases due to advances in science and medicine, it is important to understand the implications of hearing loss and how it can affect our lives.

Our bodies are amazing instruments. Hearing plays a vital role in the exchange of thoughts and ideas with others. Our ear interprets sound waves and translates them into electrical signals that the brain understands. With this connection, we can receive, process, and interact with the environment, allowing us to form strong relationships and preserve fond memories. As a result, the ear's connection to the brain can help us stay engaged and connected to those that matter most.

By using a combination of science, technology, attentive listening, and years of experience, the staff at **Prescott Hearing Center** can offer solutions that are easy to manage and of the highest value. These treatment solutions help stimulate the brain and improve mental health and cognitive function.

As a medical hearing professional, it is truly an incredible reward to help so many people achieve better hearing and communication. It is delightful to observe how a hearing aid user's attitude and personality can change dramatically in response to better hearing obtained from proper treatment. From this information, we have gained insight into how the

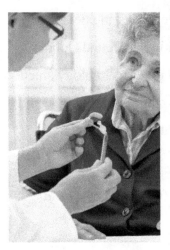

brain interacts with sound and how hearing affects health, wellness, and cognitive function. This understanding of the ear-to-brain connection makes it evident that treating hearing loss early is vital to one's overall quality of life. We take tremendous satisfaction in permanently changing people's lives.

Introduction

Being a hearing healthcare provider, hardly a day goes by when someone doesn't say, Huh? (chuckle) when responding to my profession. Yet they feel compelled to tell me that hearing treatment is not needed, as they immediately create an excuse to justify their own communication difficulties. The denial is very real for most people, but the fact is, the less you know about audiology and treating hearing loss, the more reasons there are to be afraid of it.

Many people associate hearing aids with the cumbersome, unattractive, and squealing devices that your parents or grandparents used decades ago. While using hearing aids in the past, people struggled to distinguish between speech, background noise, and other loud sounds, such as a dog barking and clattering dishes. The older technology hearing devices simply exacerbated the problem by making all sounds louder. As a result, most hearing aid users with older technology shied away from social situations, restaurants, family gatherings, and playing with grandchildren due to an outdated hearing aid.

Unfortunately, there is often a misconception that claims all hearing aids are the same and that they function as they did decades ago. Nothing could be further from the truth.

Modern small digital hearing aids present an impressive level of sophistication in their ability to process sound. These remarkable devices utilize advanced digital signal processing (DSP) algorithms to effectively distinguish and amplify specific sounds while reducing background noise. Equipped with multiple microphones, they can employ directional processing, focusing on sounds coming from a particular direction while suppressing unwanted noise from other angles. Some models even possess the capability to adapt and learn from the user's preferences and environments, adjusting their settings automatically for optimal listening experiences. With wireless connectivity, these hearing aids can seamlessly integrate with smartphones and other devices, enabling users to fine-tune settings, stream audio directly, and even receive software updates. The miniaturized hardware and cutting-edge software empower these small digital hearing aids to significantly improve the quality of life for individuals with hearing impairment.

Fear of the unknown is one reason many people hesitate to visit a hearing healthcare provider despite the abundant lifetime benefits to be gained from proper hearing healthcare. If people understood how restoring the link between the ear and the brain could help maintain their autonomy and prevent cognitive disorders, such as dementia, they might be more confident about taking this crucial step.

Patients often wait up to seven years before receiving treatment for hearing loss, a delay that can have a tremendous impact on their lives. Dementia is a particularly detrimental mental disease, as it robs individuals of their faculties and is strongly affecting an increasingly larger portion of our population. Every three to four seconds, another individual is diagnosed with dementia. It is estimated there will be a threefold increase in rates of diagnosed dementia over the next thirty years. Additionally, it is estimated that caring for a dementia patient can cost a family upwards of $57,000.00 annually. Fortunately, the treatment of hearing loss is a very important strategy toward avoiding dementia, according to a study published in *The Lancet* journal. Although a cure does not exist for this debilitating disease, there are ways to minimize its risk.

Part 1

Beginning Your Hearing Care Journey

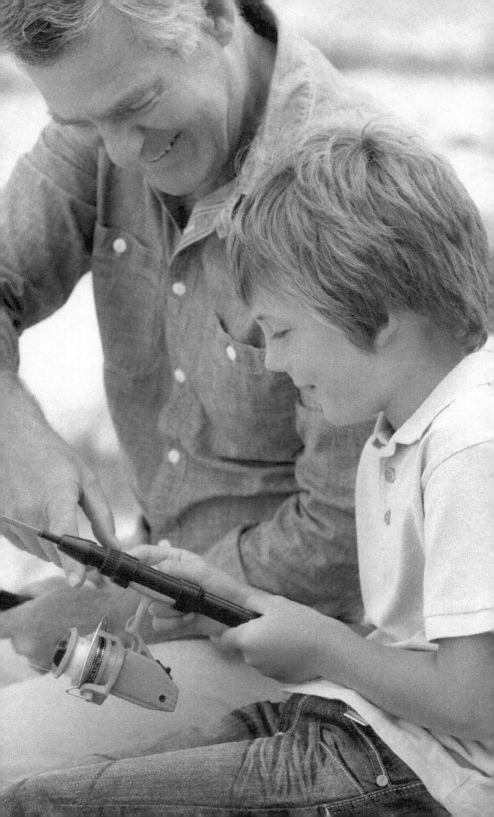

QUESTION #1

Why is hearing so important?

The ability to communicate with others or understand our surroundings depends on our hearing. Without the ability to hear, it would be difficult to process sound or understand language and develop cognitive function. Hearing also provides insight into others' emotions and experiences to help us identify when someone needs assistance. However, one of the most essential factors of hearing is the ability to protect ourselves from danger. Another less commonly known aspect of hearing is how listening to music enhances cognitive functions. Finally, hearing can help us interact with others by enhancing a more socially active lifestyle.

Communication is essential to developing and nurturing our relationships - at work, with friends, and with family. My experience working with dementia patients has given me the knowledge to better understand the connection between hearing loss and cognitive function. Our services at **Prescott Hearing Center** can now provide more enhanced care using the latest testing and treatment guidelines.

QUESTION #2

What are some early signs of hearing loss, and when should you see a hearing healthcare provider?

Hearing loss could be considered a silent disorder as it progresses slowly without pronounced symptoms. By the time someone realizes the severity, the damage could be permanent.

Common indicators might include struggling to understand speech in noisy situations, ringing in the ears (tinnitus), and feeling as though people are mumbling or speaking too softly.

People often justify hearing issues to acoustic problems in a room or business, the noise level, or how the other person is talking to them. Mild hearing loss is a significant problem if left untreated.

If someone struggles with hearing in noisy or complex listening environments, they must reflect on their communication challenges. Those with early hearing loss may find it harder to follow a conversation with multiple speakers or while at a social gathering. Often, this can cause embarrassment and lead to withdrawal from conversations, relationships, and events.

4

Eventually, that person may suffer from a diminished quality of life.

Maintaining an active social life with family and friends is essential; therefore, it is crucial to treat even mild hearing loss to keep the brain healthy. The comprehension of our environmental surroundings is strongly associated with our hearing ability.

The human ear is 'on call' 24 hours a day. It is impossible to simply close your ears, like closing your eyes. Both memory and comprehension are active functions of our brain commonly triggered by our sense of hearing. Every area of the brain is connected to the auditory system. Our brain processes sound continuously, determining whether the sound being heard is significant, which allows us to react appropriately based on how that sound was classified and remembered.

Studies from Johns Hopkins Medical Center and other organizations have revealed that mild hearing loss can raise the possibility of dementia by 200%, while more severe hearing loss can potentially increase the risk by up to 500%. Cognitive stimulation is consequently limited, even with the slightest hearing deficiency, which has been linked to cognitive deterioration and dementia. Like every major medical condition, the key to successful management of the disorder is early intervention. "Catch it early and treat it early!"

QUESTION #3

What are the reasons people avoid seeing a hearing healthcare provider?

Fear: Hearing loss can be a deeply personal issue for many people. Fear of embarrassment or attention can be a major barrier to treatment.

It is important to educate and support these individuals to help them understand there is no shame in seeking help for their hearing problems. In fact, with modern technology, no one will notice a discreet hearing aid. Thankfully, as awareness increases with the benefits of hearing, fear will diminish, and more people can be confident in treating hearing loss.

Individuals with hearing loss typically wait seven years before admitting they have a problem. In some cases, a family member may need to take the initiative to schedule a visit to our office.

A delay of seven years can greatly increase the likelihood of significant damage to the auditory system, which may reduce the effectiveness of treatment. Hearing loss is a progressive degenerative disorder that requires early intervention. Therefore, the best way to maintain clarity and good hearing quality is to treat it early. It is important to understand that the condition is irreversible and there is no cure. Fortunately, with the restorative treatments available, **Prescott Hearing Center** can help the patient stay connected and even help reduce the risk of developing dementia.

Denial: Many people with hearing loss may be in denial or have delayed seeking treatment simply because they feel it is 'not a big deal.'

Unfortunately, untreated hearing loss can have serious long-term repercussions if not addressed quickly. The effects can interfere with daily activities. There are various solutions and treatments available to help individuals, so delaying treatment should not be an option.

Others avoid getting their hearing loss treated because they deny there is an issue, even though deep down inside, they know the problem exists. Instead, they use excuses like, "I do pretty good for my age," "If people would not talk so fast," or "Some people just mumble." This may lead to confusion while trying to comprehend speech, and the frustration of misunderstanding can be significant. Fortunately, treating hearing loss for these people can be life-changing and empowering once they discover they don't have to suffer in silence.

Cost: Cost is another factor pertaining to avoidance of treating hearing loss. Higher-end hearing aids may range from several hundred dollars to more than several thousand dollars.

However, treatment for hearing loss goes far beyond the initial cost of the hearing aid. Treating hearing loss requires more time spent with the hearing healthcare professional for maintenance, checkups, and follow-ups. Investing in hearing aids may also result in additional costs for batteries, accessories, and any necessary repairs. If subjected to those costs at the initial purchase, it may seem like an exorbitant amount, but paying for every office visit for future care can get expensive too.

Hearing care professionals face many challenges when dealing with insurance companies or their intermediaries for hearing aid coverage. Unfavorable reimbursement rates and restrictive limits on the number of appointments may make it difficult to provide adequate care to the patient. Furthermore, when buying a hearing aid through an insurance plan, some patients may end up paying more than if they go directly to a hearing care provider. Rarely are other supplies and services included by your insurance company. These services may include cleaning and checks, annual adjustments, loaners, retubing, receivers, handling services, ear couplers, wax guards, counseling, and ear cleanings.

More importantly, the cost of not treating hearing loss, although difficult to measure, is likely much more significant. The side effects of untreated hearing loss may include a diminished comfort level in social situations and higher levels of stress, anxiety, and depression. Other long-term problems that accompany untreated hearing loss may include difficulty paying attention, leading to decreased quality of life, increased risk of falling, and cognitive decline.

Investing in hearing aids and follow-up care can help ensure that one's hearing and quality of life are protected. Ultimately, the cost of not treating hearing loss may likely be much more than the cost of proper treatment.

No One Wants A Hearing Aid: Let's face it, hearing aids are not the most desirable worldly possessions. Nor is acknowledging a hearing loss at the top of our list of joys to celebrate. The idea of having to wear a hearing aid for the remainder of one's life is discouraging and may be hard to accept. Individuals may be familiar with a companion who owns hearing aids but doesn't use them or have memories of

Grandpa's hearing aid that gave an irritating screech when you hugged him 40 years ago. Furthermore, fear of discomfort or not liking anything in your ears can pose an obstacle. In many cases, hearing aids are perceived as unsightly, giving them an unpleasant appearance and attracting unwanted attention. In addition, there is a stigma attached to the use of hearing aids as being a sign of sickness, advancing age, or physical or mental condition.

Although hearing aids may have all the above stigmas, it is important to know these negative viewpoints are not aligned with reality. Remember, hearing aids are a critical device for those with significant hearing loss to live a more normal life. They can help improve hearing-related quality of life, boost self-confidence, and bring social, psychological, and physical benefits. Additionally, with advances in technology, hearing aids are becoming increasingly comfortable, discreet, and effective. Therefore, the benefits outweigh the drawbacks, and it is important for people with hearing loss to get the help they need.

QUESTION #4

How should I choose a hearing healthcare provider?

The following items are important to consider before choosing a hearing healthcare provider.

1. *Does the specialist have a great reputation?*

The internet makes it easy to search ratings and reviews of local hearing healthcare providers. Moreover, do not hesitate to ask for references from a hearing healthcare office. Or talk with other individuals about their hearing providers.

2. *Does the office and staff make you feel special and comfortable?*

At **Prescott Hearing Center**, we want patients to feel comfortable and welcome when receiving hearing health care. We understand that managing hearing loss and the decision to get help can be a source of stress or sadness. Therefore, the atmosphere in our office is aimed at relieving anxiousness. Our staff's priority is to ensure every patient feels the respect they deserve. All patients should receive the highest quality of care possible.

3. Does the specialist think brain first?

Most people believe that their hearing is solely dependent on their ears when in truth, it is the brain that processes sound. Modern treatments are far more sophisticated than 'amplifiers' behind the ears.

If a hearing healthcare provider does not prioritize the brain in their treatment plan, it might be wise to get a second opinion. Treatments should help restore lost clarity, provide noise-canceling capabilities, and amplify soft speech for those with low voices. The cost of untreated hearing loss could be catastrophic for a patient.

4. Do they include a free demonstration after diagnostics are completed?

While there is no right or wrong answer here, you must consider a hearing aid demonstration's real purpose and benefit. For someone without an idea of what amplification may sound like, it may be a pleasant experience to relieve some apprehension the new user may be experiencing. However, if the demonstration is used to determine the full performance of the hearing aids, it may be difficult to surmise their full capabilities with a quick demonstration.

If the amplification is perceived as too loud, the user may immediately reject the hearing aid as 'noisy.' However, if the amplification is turned down to a comfortable level, the benefits may be limited at the onset, and treatment could be rejected due to the perceived poor performance. Therefore, it is somewhat unfair to all parties involved in passing judgment based on a brief demonstration. Instead, consider the trial period of the provider as a true test of the performance of the devices. Our office offers a sixty-day return privilege since we believe that is enough time to demonstrate the performance of the instruments and allow the user to get fully adapted to them.

5. *Does the hearing healthcare provider offer an evaluation period with a comprehensive treatment plan?*

Many discount providers, big-box stores, and insurance plan providers focus on the hearing aids themselves without taking into consideration the personalized needs of the patient. A personalization plan should include the physical, psychological, and cognitive abilities of the patient. For example, a narrow and twisted ear canal can sound significantly different than one larger and straight. The seemingly simple coupling of the hearing aid to the user's ear can play a major role in the success of a hearing aid fitting. Consistently following a proven treatment plan will help ensure the user's success and acceptance of the new devices.

6. *Is he or she ensuring you are properly fitted by verification and validation?*

Verifying the hearing aid response using real ear measurements is essential to ensure adequate auditory stimulation. Background noise testing before and after fitting patients with hearing aids should be completed to ensure the technology is being used properly. The highest level of performance is necessary so the patient can achieve the benefits. Other pre- and post-fitting measures will also demonstrate the value of properly fitted hearing aids.

7. *Does your provider explain all the details of your treatment plan?*

Our goal at **Prescott Hearing Center** is for all patients to understand the treatment plan from day one. Many patients are unaware of the treatment process and expect a single visit will be satisfactory to resolve their long-term needs for hearing healthcare. When they discover the need for follow-up appointments to maximize the benefits and gain a full appreciation of how the instruments function, they understand the purpose of a properly designed and implemented treatment plan going forward. Periodic cleaning of the hearing aids, office visits, and prescriptive programming will be needed throughout the life of the product.

8. *Does the specialist charge for follow-up visits and supplies?*

Again, there is no right or wrong answer to this question, but a seemingly competitive price for hearing aids is often at the sacrifice of follow-up treatment and supplies. The cost of this ongoing treatment should be considered while the purchase is being made. All patients should be educated on what services are provided in the treatment care plan.

QUESTION #5

How early in life should I have my hearing evaluated?

- The Simple Answer

Anyone ages fifty and older should have their hearing evaluated.

- Detailed Answer

The importance of early treatment for hearing loss is essential to minimize any long-term problems.

> According to the American Medical Association (AMA), "People should check their hearing if they experience prolonged hearing or balance issues, such as sudden or gradual hearing loss, constant ringing in the ears, vertigo, or are exposed to loud noises regularly."

A baseline hearing test can be helpful to ensure a primary care doctor knows of any underlying issues. Not only can it serve as a reference to guide medical decisions down the line, but it can also provide reassurance that your hearing is healthy if the test results show normal hearing. Unfortunately, waiting too long can significantly impact the expectations and outcome of treatment. Sadly, every hearing healthcare clinician I know has a patient who waited too long for treatment, of which, unfortunately, the benefits of treatment will be minimal.

Part 2

Understanding the Problem

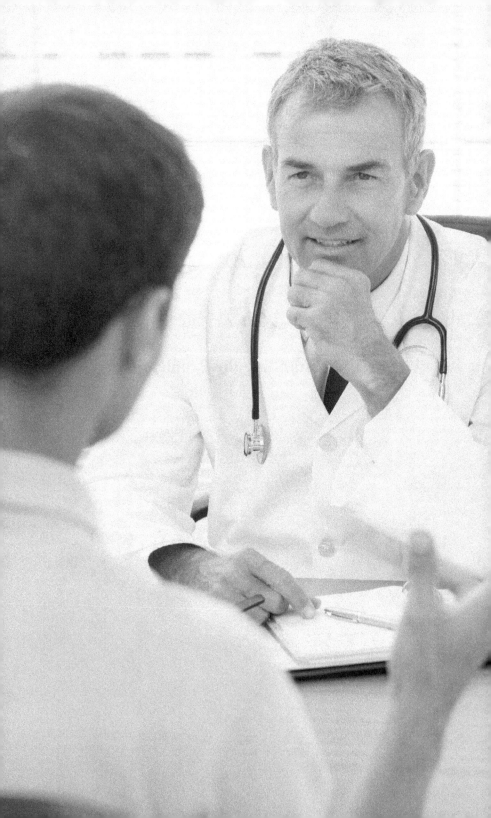

QUESTION #6

What will happen during the initial evaluation and consultation?

Getting to know the patient is a critical first step during the initial evaluation. One of the first questions you will hear from me is, *"Tell me, what is going on with your ears?"*

This question helps evaluate specific hearing-related issues, concerns, and experiences. Your responses provide a baseline to help the clinician understand 'why' the reason for your visit.

One part of elevated health care pertains to understanding a patient at a deeper, more emotional level. As a hearing clinician, I take great pride in getting to know more about my patient's lives. Some very important areas of life can be greatly affected by hearing loss.

Treating hearing loss is a process immersed in science, engineering, and technology. There is also an 'art' to treating hearing loss–a skill that takes years to develop. The process begins with a proper diagnosis.

Overview of how the ear works.

Before treating any patient, it is important to review the process and help them understand how the ear works. The ear collects acoustic sound waves (all the sounds around us travel in invisible sound waves) and turns them into electrical signals for our nervous system and brain to interpret.

When a sound is made, acoustical energy vibrates the eardrum and converts the sound waves into mechanical energy. Attached to the eardrum are a series of tiny bones that move to transmit energy into the inner ear, also known as the cochlea.

The cochlea organ is located inside the temporal bone, which is the densest bone of the human body. Its size is only slightly bigger than a fingernail bed! Within the inner ear, this mechanical energy changes to hydraulic energy, as it produces a current throughout the fluid. The current causes hairlike "hair cells" inside the cochlea to move in a manner similar to how seaweed sways in ocean currents. Lastly, the hydraulic energy is changed to electrical energy, which is then conducted through the eighth cranial nerve and sent to the auditory centers of the brain. The characteristic of the sound is distinguished by the electrical

Figure 1 Cochlea Organ

22

energy to the brain; this method helps the brain interpret and process speech even with the presence of background noise. And this all happens in milliseconds!

The assessment

It is essential that the healthcare professional accurately identifies the source of any hearing problem. During the assessment, the provider shall analyze the various stages of sound transmission to determine if there is a loss of energy at any point. When this is established, we can identify if the issue is earwax, middle ear damage, or damage to the inner ear hair cells. If earwax is the culprit, it can be easily removed. However, a middle ear issue may be treatable through medical intervention. If the inner ear hair cells are at fault, additional sound stimulation may be needed.

Hearing care professionals will start by examining the ear canal to ensure it is free of any obstructing cerumen (ear wax). Often, a procedure follows the process called *tympanometry*, which can rule out any medical condition causing hearing loss, including the eardrum and/or the space behind it, including those tiny middle ear bones.

The Beeps

Hearing loss is measured by a ranking from stage 0 to stage 4. The patient will push a button when a 'beep' is heard. By performing this test, the provider can vary the level of sound. As fundamental as this may seem, it serves a valuable purpose in establishing the degree of hearing loss.

The Words

The most important testing we will perform is designed to assess your cognitive hearing, e.g., how well you understand words in quiet and with background noise. After all, nobody comes to the office complaining they can't hear beeps!

The term word discrimination refers to the patient's ability to understand spoken language. A patient is asked to repeat a set of words presented at a near-normal conversational volume. Those with normal hearing ability usually repeat 96 to 100% of what was said. In contrast, an individual with hearing loss will have a lower score - it may be as low as 50-60% or below. It is a difficult conversation with the patient because they miss 40-50% of the words spoken daily. Unfortunately, if they do not have visual or contextual cues to support what was said, the meaning of the interaction is lost.

The next test is a repeat, almost exactly as just described, but performed at a volume and clarity setting ideal for the specific patient's hearing loss. The result of this second round of word testing is referred to as the patient's "Hearing Potential Score." The patient's score should show considerable improvement and give us a predictable outcome with our treatment plan. Not only is the patient fully aware of their performance improvement, but they also realize the reduced effort that was expended compared to the first time the test was performed.

However, when scores of the second test do not improve, there is a much bleaker prognosis. I mentioned earlier that the consequences of ignoring hearing loss can be dire. In some cases, when the second round of word testing is completed, the patient's "Hearing Potential Score" will be nearly the same as the original score. While hearing aids may offer a limited amount of benefit, the neurological damage may have already progressed to a point where the desired outcomes may not be achieved with traditional treatment.

The words in background noise

In almost every case, the number one complaint of hearing loss is the patient's difficulty understanding speech and conversation in the presence of background noise. Therefore, the clinician needs to assess the patient's ability to decipher speech in background noise without any visual or contextual help.

Speech in noise testing is intended to start easy and progressively become more difficult as the background babble gets louder. We find the threshold where speech is still understood with the highest level of background noise as SNR-50. The number represents the difference in intensity between the speech and background noise. As in golf, the lower number represents a better score.

Individuals with normal hearing typically grade at SNR-50 levels less than 3 decibels. Patients with mild hearing loss can struggle significantly on this test when the noise is 10 decibels less. The test is scored on a Hearing Handicap Scale ranging from normal, mild, moderate, or severe.

The results

Results of testing should be shared with the patient and anyone else at their request. Once the tests are reviewed, the clinician can make recommendations as to the next steps, depending on the outcome.

When a patient is given troubling news about their hearing difficulties, the diagnosis can be devastating news to them and their family. Yet finding out the potential benefits of treatment can quickly encourage a patient to take decisive action to potentially prevent the more challenging outcomes of not treating hearing loss, which may significantly change their quality of life.

QUESTION #7

What if I still have questions after the initial consultation?

The initial consultation, including the diagnosis of hearing loss, can seem overwhelming for the patient and their loved ones. Therefore, it is important to maintain an open dialog with the hearing healthcare provider to help minimize any concerns about treatment options.

Your hearing care provider should be able to guide you to the resources you need to understand hearing loss and treatment options so that you feel comfortable during your hearing healthcare journey.

At **Prescott Hearing Center**, we always welcome and encourage our patients to bring loved ones to their appointments.

QUESTION #8

When is the best time to treat my hearing loss?

As with any health diagnosis, treatment should be considered and applied as soon as possible. The negative effects left untreated can have substantial impacts on your health.

The extent of hearing loss dictates the treatment plan. It could include hearing aids, learning listening strategies, or trying new assistive technology. An early diagnosis and treatment plan can help preserve communication abilities and improve hearing and speech development.

Auditory Deprivation

It is important to understand auditory deprivation, otherwise known as sound deprivation. Hearing loss can impact cognitive development functions, causing problems in comprehension, lowering memory recognition, decreasing creativity, and greater stress levels. When our ability to communicate effectively is reduced, self-expression, socializing, and emotional development can also be affected. When hearing loss is left untreated, it can cause an overload of information.

In neuroscience, this is called '*Cognitive Overload.*' The brain is asked to process auditory, visual, and other cues to put together a simple sentence.

Consider this sentence:

Hi Martha! How is your puppy doing? Is he eating and growing okay? I hope we can get our dogs together soon to play.

If we filter this sentence through a typical mild age-related hearing loss with compromised clarity (e.g., difficulty hearing consonants), the sentence could be perceived as this:

i Mara! ow i our uy oing? I e eaing and groing o a? I ope e an ge our do ogeer oon o ay.

The result is rather alarming. In a normal conversational volume, patients with mild hearing loss missing 50-60% of words could hear the sentence, as illustrated above. Of course, the brain will use visual cues, lip-reading, etc., to fill in the missing pieces. The brain was not designed to take on that much stress to understand a simple sentence.

Cognitive overload is a leading reason why individuals with hearing loss are five times more likely to develop dementia.

QUESTION #9

What if I am nervous about treating my hearing loss?

Technology has advanced extensively, allowing any patient to enjoy the benefits of wearing hearing aids discreetly. The fit is comfortable and can be worn all day without difficulty. Most people discover the process is less intimidating than originally perceived.

The enhanced clarity features, background noise cancellation filters, and wireless connectivity make today's hearing loss treatment options simple and often a fun experience that makes life easier instead of more complicated.

Our goal is to provide a treatment that will fit well, feel good, and, of course, 'sound good.' The journey to better hearing health should be a comfortable experience, delivered in a timely fashion that is appropriate for each individual.

QUESTION #10

Can I wait to treat my hearing loss?

People often delay treatment of hearing loss for various reasons. The most common reason, in my experience, is that the one suffering from hearing loss is unaware of the extent of auditory damage with which they are living. Others may be concerned with cost or committing to long-term hearing aid maintenance. Patients have also shown concern over potential lifestyle limitations.

In many cases, even when these obstacles are addressed, hearing loss is often rationalized by insisting, 'This is normal for my age' or 'Everybody Mumbles'. However, the consequences of ignoring hearing loss treatment can create serious health complications.

In the inner ear (cochlea), there are a finite number of receptor cells—referred to as hair cells. The progression of degeneration, while gradual, contributes to a continual loss of these hair cells within the cochlea. While the cells have upwards of 35 fibers responsible for relaying information, they are a finite number. Nerve fibers send signals to the brain, which process sounds and conversation. However, as the cells die with age and excessive exposure to noise, so do the neurons.

A more disturbing study came from Johns Hopkins linking hearing loss to dementia.

> "Quantifying hearing loss's impact. Hearing loss is estimated to account for 8% of dementia cases. This means hearing loss may be responsible for 800,000 of the nearly 10 million new cases of dementia diagnosed each year."

> "Hearing loss has long-term effects on health. It is believed to increase the risk of falls and depression. It also leads to higher health care costs: People with hearing loss have, over ten years, a 47% increased rate of hospitalization."

The study determined significant cerebral atrophy (AKA brain shrinkage) in the brains of individuals with hearing loss.

As these studies proved, early treatment for hearing loss is essential to limiting the damage caused by ignoring the problem. The adage '*Use It or Lose It*' comes immediately to mind. Although treating hearing loss cannot prevent further damage caused by genetics or prior exposure to loud noise, it can help maintain clarity of speech as the disorder progresses.

The ability to strengthen neural connections is key to successfully treating hearing loss.

Studies show that untreated ear performance of word discrimination tasks is significantly reduced compared to the treated ear. However, even in light of this evidence, people still neglect treatment.

In the event a hearing test shows damage in both ears, the treatment should also reflect the diagnosis. It is important to treat hearing loss in both ears to prevent further damage, maintain balance, and provide increased sound localization and clarity. The treatment can also include relief from tinnitus symptoms. Ignoring the hearing loss in just one ear can cause sound distortion, which will diminish hearing in the good ear over time, resulting in increased damage.

Part 3

Focusing on a Plan That Works for You

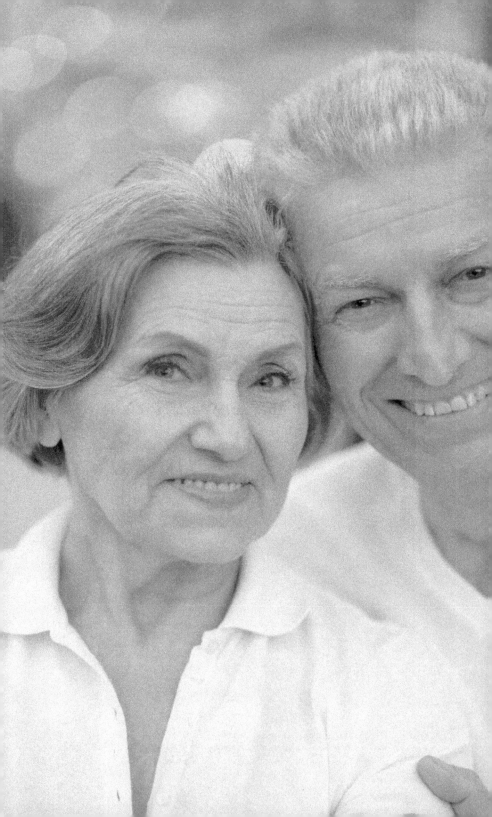

QUESTION #11

Who is the ideal patient?

Ideal patients are aware that medical and personal implications can arise if treatment is avoided. In the same context, hearing loss not only affects the individual but also affects family, coworkers, and friends.

When someone pursues treatment, they can invest in living life to the fullest, maintaining independence, being connected in part of a conversation, and staying central to family life and the local community.

In my professional opinion, it is difficult to put a dollar value on improved health. The cost-benefit ratio is incalculable. However, not all patients want to consider treating hearing loss. Many of them are pushed into visiting a clinician to determine what problems might exist. Nevertheless, the patient must ultimately make the final decision.

QUESTION #12

What treatment options are available for my hearing loss?

The most common types of hearing aids include:

1. Receiver-In-The-Canal (RIC): RIC hearing aids are a combination of BTE and CIC hearing aids. A tiny receiver is placed inside the ear canal, with the microphone, amplifier, and power supply of the device worn behind the ear.

2. In-The-Ear (ITE): ITE hearing aids are composed of a shell that fits inside the outer ear.

3. Behind-The-Ear (BTE): BTE hearing aids are secured behind the ear with a tube that connects to a customized mold in the ear canal.

4. Completely-In-The-Canal (CIC): CIC hearing aids are designed to fit completely in the ear canal.

5. Invisible-In-The-Canal (IIC): IIC hearing aids are custom-made and fit deep into the ear canals, making them nearly invisible. This technology is intended for maximum discreteness.

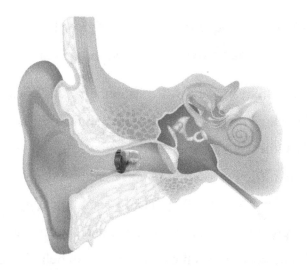

All hearing aids have various options. Some perform better than others, depending on the situation. The style of hearing aids includes size, design, and type of technology,

In most cases, smaller hearing aids generally provide variable acoustic performance by blocking ambient sound that would otherwise go directly into the ear canal. The feature may improve or degrade sound clarity and fidelity depending on the type and severity of the hearing loss.

Also, modern hearing aids are equipped with sophisticated digital signal processing (DSP) software to improve sound quality. The technology can detect and amplify weak signals while compressing louder sounds by reducing background noises. In addition, some hearing aid models are designed to target specific sound frequencies, such as high or low frequencies, which may provide additional sound clarity.

Hearing healthcare providers will consider a patient's hearing profile and medical history when recommending specific hearing aids. Other factors, such as the patient's symptoms (including any difficulty hearing in noisy environments, tinnitus, etc.), dexterity (can they handle a small hearing aid?), and personal preferences in terms of style and size, are also considered. The hearing healthcare provider can help the patient understand which hearing aid style, shape, size, and features will provide the best solution and optimize them for peak performance.

QUESTION #13

What treatment options are available for the ringing in my ears (aka tinnitus)?

One of the most common issues for patients with hearing loss is 'ringing' in the ears. *Tinnitus*, which is pronounced either TIH·nih· tus or tuh·NYE· tus, is defined as a sensation of sound in a person's ears or head. However, everyone's experience with tinnitus is different. It is usually described as a ringing sound, but can also be referred to as a shooshing, static, buzzing, or whooshing sound, like a conch shell.

Tinnitus may be extremely distressing, but not all hope is lost. Although tinnitus cannot be cured, it can be managed effectively to help the patient. One relatively successful method is the use of hearing aids fitted to both ears, as this helps the brain become less aware of ear ringing.

According to the National Institute on Deafness and Other Communication Disorders (NIDCD), "An estimated 50 million adults in the United States have some form of tinnitus. Tinnitus is experienced by approximately 80% of people living with hearing loss. Around half of those people also report hearing loss."

Tinnitus should never be overlooked; it could point to an internal alarm about something more serious. Tinnitus may not be constant, for example, heard only in a quiet room or at night, pulsating, or triggered by certain activities, such as exercising or drinking caffeine. To fully assess the condition and implement an effective treatment plan, it is critical to seek proper hearing healthcare and advice from your medical doctor. Tinnitus could also be a sign of issues such as depression, anxiety, concentration trouble, and sleep disruption, as well as negative thoughts and emotions.

What is the cause of tinnitus?

The primary reason for tinnitus is damage to the auditory organ, the cochlea, which is analogous to the eyes in the sense of vision. The cochlea contains fragile hair cells, and once these are hurt, the nerves that link the hair cells to the brain (responsible for allowing us to hear) are irreversibly harmed; subsequently, a loud ringing sound appears.

How Do the Sensory Cells in My Ear Get Damaged?

Sensory cells in the ear can be damaged due to loud noises, head trauma, certain medications, infections, and aging.

Exposure to loud noises, such as concerts or loud machinery, can damage the delicate sensory cells in the inner ear and lead to hearing loss or tinnitus. Similarly, a hard strike to the head can also damage these cells. Medications, such as high doses of certain antibiotics and chemotherapy agents, can also do damage to the inner ear sensory cells. Infections in the inner ear, such as meningitis or a virus, can cause damage to these cells, leading to hearing damage or deafness. Lastly, aging can cause the delicate sensory cells in the inner ear to break down, leading to a decreased ability to hear.

But Why Do My Ears Ring?

Its cause is thought to stem from a phenomenon called central gain, where auditory stimulation is decreased due to some degree of hearing impairment. The response is similar to a phantom limb, in which the brain compensates for an alteration in the peripheral nervous system, such as an amputation, by releasing pain signals. In tinnitus, the perceived discomfort is a continuous ringing sound in the ear.

Is there a Treatment for My Tinnitus?

Unfortunately, many patients have been told nothing can be done, however, this isn't the case. There are clinical treatment solutions proven to help mitigate, and sometimes even fully resolve, tinnitus symptoms.

Hearing treatment plans are the most effective treatment option available for patients suffering from tinnitus. The FDA has approved a treatment that provides the brain with restored and proper brain stimulus. Furthermore, new hearing technology helps people with hearing loss, as well as those with 'normal' hearing. A myriad of studies suggests that those who use hearing aid technology observe a sharp decrease in their tinnitus, with some even claiming that 'the ringing is gone all day.'

QUESTION #14

What if I have total hearing loss in one of my ears? And what is a CROS System?

Generally speaking, both ears should possess a near-equal hearing capacity since they are the same age. If there was previous exposure to loud noises, it probably affected both ears in the same way. Moreover, if you took medications with auditory side effects, both ears were likely impacted in the same manner.

Some patients can experience differences in hearing levels between their right and left ears caused by various otologic issues, such as a viral infection, physical trauma, or unknown (idiopathic) hearing loss. These discrepancies can range from mild to severe and can even lead to complete deafness (anacusis) in one ear while the other ear remains unaffected. Asymmetric hearing loss is also common, which occurs when one ear has a more serious hearing loss than the other.

Humans are designed to listen through two ears (binaural) for a reason. Binaural hearing allows someone to pinpoint the direction of sound and better understand speech in a noisy setting. The benefit of hearing with two ears is known as the 'Binaural Advantage.' If you know someone with a hearing deficiency that manifests as lopsided hearing, they usually adjust their surroundings so the speaker is on the side where they can hear better.

Those who suffer greater hearing loss in one ear may have an alternative treatment than those with an even deficit in both ears. The hearing healthcare provider can put together a plan of action to optimize hearing comprehension, regardless of the circumstances.

A CROS (Contralateral Routing of Signal) hearing device is a type of hearing aid designed to pick up sound from one ear and transmit it to the other. The device consists of two parts: a transmitting unit, worn on the poorer hearing ear, and a receiver, worn on the better hearing ear. The transmitting unit collects sound from its environment, which is then processed and sent to the receiver. The receiver then amplifies the sound and delivers it to the better-hearing ear.

The results help improve understanding of speech or other sounds that would be unclear to the user without the device. While this patient may never perform as well as an individual treating equal levels of hearing loss in both ears, restoring the perception of sound from the muted side of the body can offer significant relief in almost all listening situations.

QUESTION #15

What is an over-the-counter (OTC) hearing aid, and would it work for me?

An over-the-counter hearing aid is a type of hearing device or hearing aid that does not require a prescription and can be purchased off the shelf. These hearing aids are compact and typically cost less than prescription hearing aids. A small battery usually powers them and contains a microphone, an amplifier, and a loudspeaker. The microphone detects sound and amplifies it, while the loudspeaker transmits amplified sound waves directly into the ear canal. They typically come with features such as volume control and feedback dampening but usually lack more advanced features common in prescription hearing aids.

Many people ask, "Would they work for me?"

My response would be, "I don't know, maybe."

A patient would never know the true benefits or shortcomings of an over-the-counter hearing aid either. While these devices may help improve the perceived hearing ability of some individuals, they will likely fall short of desired expectations.

48

When expectations are not predefined or quantified, the outcomes are going to be ambiguous at best. Simply making sounds louder might seem like an appropriate step, but the negative consequences of over or under-amplification may prove more detrimental overall.

Some frequencies may be over-amplified, and other frequencies may be totally missed. The repercussions of a poorly fitted hearing aid may be as bad as no hearing aid at all or may be so disappointing to the user that he or she decides not to seek additional help for even longer since hearing aids obviously 'don't work.'

These devices are symbolic of the old 'beige bananas' that Grandpa used to wear 30 to 40 years ago. This older technology was intended to make sounds louder regardless of location in the room, the volume of the incoming sounds, and whether the patient even wanted to hear the sound.

QUESTION #16

Do hearing aids really work?

The advancement of technology has significantly benefited hearing aid manufacturing, by which miniature devices, better circuits, microphones, and receivers allow hearing aids to become much more powerful and reliable. New technology has also enabled the ability to customize hearing aids to individual needs. Plus, sophisticated, user-friendly devices can be adjusted easily through simple buttons and settings on a smartphone or computer.

> "Ten years ago, the satisfaction rate for hearing aid users was reportedly around 79%. Today, it is estimated to be around 86%.

> "The stats show a higher satisfaction rate than that of smartphones, which the American Customer Satisfaction Index reports at 81%."

Hearing aids today provide users with an exceptional hearing experience that exceeds their expectations.

Advanced hearing technology is designed to enhance hearing in all listening situations, increase clarity of speech details, and automatically provide an increased boost of volume for soft speakers while stimulating the brain and increasing cognitive function. What's not to like?

QUESTION #17

What advanced technology is available for treating hearing loss?

Modern hearing aids contain digital signal processing (DSP) technology, which is highly advanced, offering users adjustments to sound in an unprecedented manner.

The six main features of a digital hearing aid are noise reduction, amplified sound, frequency compression, automatic programs, wireless technology, and rechargeable batteries.

Noise Reduction - Noise reduction technology filters out background noises and optimizes the signal so the user can better understand and focus on what they are hearing. The hearing aid differentiates specific sound patterns between speech and background noise, making it easier for the user to hear and understand speech. For people who struggle with environmental noise, this feature can be invaluable.

Amplified Sound – Many digital hearing aids offer personalized sound amplification tailored to the user's needs. Digital hearing aids use a computer-controlled system to adjust sound levels automatically, making sure the user can hear at natural sound levels.

Frequency Compression – Modern hearing aids compress sound for hearing-impaired individuals, making things audible. The technology is designed to maximize the amount of information heard by users.

Automatic Programs - Digital hearing aids often come with various preset programs applied to sound by a sound classification system. For instance, the hearing aid will respond to diverse environmental noises, such as speech in quiet, speech in noise, traffic, music, or outdoor sounds. It can also modify the microphone configuration and frequency response to optimize sound quality without any user input, as the hearing aid registers the attributes of the sound.

Wireless Technology - Some digital hearing aids have wireless connectivity, allowing them to pair with Bluetooth devices such as telephones or MP3 players. The feature allows the user to wirelessly stream sound signals directly into their hearing aids.

Rechargeable batteries – Patients can eliminate the need to constantly purchase, store, and replace traditional batteries. It also makes it more convenient, as the battery can be recharged at any time with a charging station. Rechargeable batteries last longer than traditional batteries, saving money overall.

These features clearly show the need for digital hearing aids as a viable solution for hearing-impaired patients. The user can customize sound and filter out background noise, allowing the customization of their sound experience according to preferences. The use of wireless technology allows users to experience the joys of sound and live an easier life.

Part 4

Financing Your Hearing Loss Treatment Without Breaking the Bank

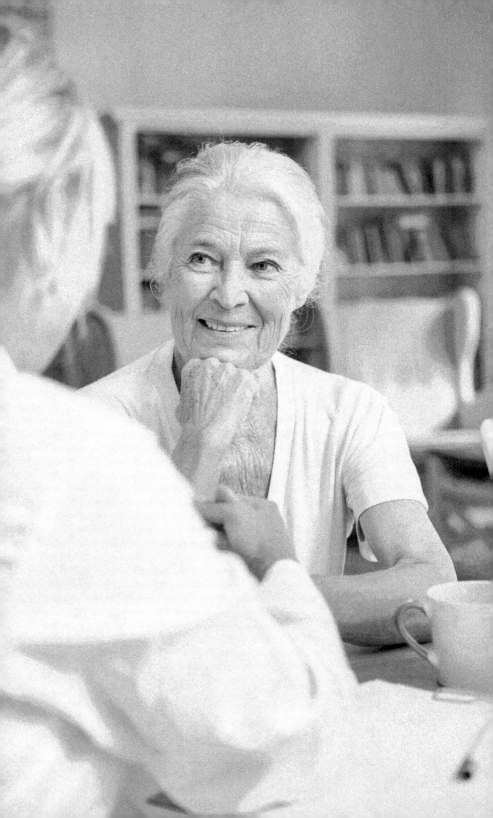

QUESTION #18

How much will my "new ears" cost me?

Answer: It depends.

The cost of hearing treatment varies greatly, depending on the type of treatment and severity of the hearing loss. In other words, treating the progressive degenerative nature of age-related hearing loss is no different than treating other major medical disorders as you age.

Picture a situation where you or a loved one needed hip replacement surgery. Could you imagine your surgeon asking the following question?

"Would you like me to replace your hip and restore 50%, 70%, or maximum mobility?"

Here is another example: Imagine saying to your heart surgeon after he or she lets you know that you are required to undergo triple bypass and heart valve replacement:

"Doc, if you don't mind, I'm going to shop online for a replacement valve to try and save a few bucks, even if it doesn't pump the adequate amount of blood to keep my body oxygenated and healthy."

While both scenarios may seem ridiculous, unfortunately, the retail aspect of hearing health care has 'poisoned the well' for too many people. The result made treatment a very confusing and onerous process for the patient seeking hearing help.

We trust that healthcare providers will use their knowledge and expertise to provide the best, most medically sound treatment recommendation, regardless of price. You should expect the same from your hearing healthcare provider. If your clinician is reputable (e.g., is referred to by local physicians, has great reviews online, has readily available current patient liaisons to speak with, etc.), and has longevity in the community, then you can rest assured their pricing structure is standard; the only variable is the cost of technology (preset by the manufacturer).

QUESTION #19

What is the cost of not treating my hearing loss?

Answer: Possibly a lot more than you think!

Untreated hearing loss can have a significant monetary impact on individuals, families, and society. It can lead to significant economic costs due to reduced productivity and poorer quality of life.

> In a report by the National Institute of Health (NIH), "The estimated cost of untreated hearing loss in the United States is $100 billion annually."

Here are three examples relating to the fiscal implications of untreated hearing loss.

> **Example 1:** Studies have demonstrated those with untreated hearing loss may suffer financially, such as a decrease in salary and an enhanced possibility of joblessness. A yearly average of up to $12,000 in salary can be at stake. Fortunately, treatment of hearing loss may reduce these losses by up to 50%. It appears that people with hearing loss often have difficulty acquiring

and keeping jobs due to various issues, including frequent communication difficulties, limited training options, and a shortage of awareness in enterprises regarding their prospective talent. This is true for workers of all ages.

Example 2: Hearing loss can increase the risk of dementia by 200-500%. Treating hearing loss is the most effective modifiable risk factor to prevent dementia. Given these medical research findings, it is not unreasonable to calculate the cost of treating a patient with dementia that could have been avoided by treating his or her hearing loss at an earlier age. Statistics show the average family will spend approximately $57,000.00 per year to cover health care costs and manage the care of a loved one with dementia.

Example 3: Seniors with hearing loss are at increased risk of falling, which can be greatly diminished by treating the condition. Based on this fact and statistics from the Centers for Disease Control and Prevention (CDC), it makes sense to compare the cost of treating falls to treating hearing loss. Falls account for the most fatal injuries in individuals aged sixty-five and above, and survivors have a greater chance of suffering another fall in the future. The CDC reports that a fall resulting in hospitalization typically costs around $24,000. This figure increases with age.

In addition, co-morbidities of hearing loss (other diseases correlated with hearing loss) extend to diabetes, coronary disease, thyroid disease, kidney disease, and others. When we associate hearing health with general health, it is not surprising the costs associated with neglecting treatment can be astronomical.

QUESTION #20

How do I pay for my hearing healthcare?

It should be no surprise that treatment for your hearing loss can be a considerable investment. Like any major medical procedure, audiology can cost several thousand dollars, and insurance may not cover all the expenses, depending on your plan. However, affordable options for treatment are available, with some of the options listed below:

Flexible Spending Account (FSA)

A Flexible Spending Account (FSA) can provide a great way to cover the costs of hearing aids. Some advantages of using an FSA may include pre-tax contributions, which generally allow individuals to use the account funds immediately, and up to a $2,750 annual allowance typically provided by FSAs in most states. Additionally, depending on an employer's rules, an FSA may cover both the cost of the hearing aid and required batteries or accessories. The cost can likely be spread over multiple paychecks.

Financing

Medical financing is often a cost-effective method to provide funding. In return, the payments can be divided over several months or years. Since financing is available in many forms, check with your hearing healthcare provider for options.

- Same as cash financing
- Term loan through a bank or credit union
- Down payment with monthly payments
- 0% cash advance on a credit card

Selling unneeded items

Often, people have valuable collectibles that could be sold for additional cash. A gold coin, jewelry, or a neglected boat in the garage are all common examples. The ability to upgrade your quality of life with improved hearing will have an even greater impact than you can imagine.

Getting a part-time job

Many people often retire due to hearing loss but secretly want to keep working. The benefits of maintaining your hearing ability through the use of hearing aids can greatly enhance your quality of life. You could even confidently return to work part-time to help pay for them.

Reverse mortgage

A reverse mortgage can be a great way to access funds to pay for hearing aids. It essentially allows seniors to borrow against the equity in their homes. The benefits of eliminating mortgage payments do not only allow the purchase of hearing aids but also decrease the stress of high monthly costs.

The benefits may also allow tax-free incentives on the money seniors borrow, with some reverse mortgage packages. Ironically, hearing aids might let the borrower stay at home longer than if the hearing loss was left untreated.

When there is a will, there is a way.

Being able to differentiate between necessities and luxuries is an important skill. It is especially significant when someone is dealing with hearing loss, as it is necessary for them to invest in treatment. Fortunately, once the priority is set, the reward of improved auditory and cognitive capabilities more than offsets the cost.

QUESTION #21

Does my insurance cover the cost of hearing treatment?

Short answer: That depends.

As science reveals a growing connection between hearing loss and its effects on health, insurance companies are showing increased interest in hearing healthcare coverage. However, because health insurance coverage is an intricate and constantly fluctuating set of regulations, there is no one-size-fits-all answer when it comes to determining one's coverage.

After years of providing patient care and working with many different insurance companies, we have discovered that there are typically three distinct offerings when it comes to hearing healthcare offered through an insurance company.

- Insurance companies may offer a 'dollar benefit' that applies to the cost of your hearing treatment.
- Insurance companies may work with a third-party facilitator to offer a 'discount plan.'
- Insurance companies provide the hearing aid directly or through a contracted provider.

Insurance companies may provide a predetermined amount of dollars to be spent on hearing healthcare. Typically, the benefit can be applied directly to the cost of the devices or services within the limits of the plan. Of course, these amounts may be subject to coinsurance and plan deductibles, but usually, this is the most straightforward in terms of receiving a quantifiable benefit.

When considering the purchase of hearing aids, some people find the prospect of buying hearing aids directly from an insurance company or through a third-party administrator an attractive option. However, when it comes to finding the necessary treatment and care, patients may encounter limitations on the type of device, care, or location where the treatment can be received. In some cases, purchasing directly from the insurance company may be more expensive than going directly to the provider of the patient's choice. These restrictions can greatly reduce the quality of the treatment you may expect to receive.

When insurance companies limit the offering of products or services to the members of their plan, it can be difficult for providers to participate with these companies in good faith. Sacrificing quality of care or product preference can make it an ethical dilemma for providers who choose to offer best practices to their patients.

In conclusion, it is best to ensure that healthcare decisions stay with the patient. You should always have the choice for all your medical treatment options. Avoid situations that give the insurance company the power to make those decisions for you. A good hearing healthcare provider should always explain your options on coverage and out-of-pocket expenses and whether your insurance company is offering the best solution for you.

Part 5

Treating Hearing Loss & Your Overall Health

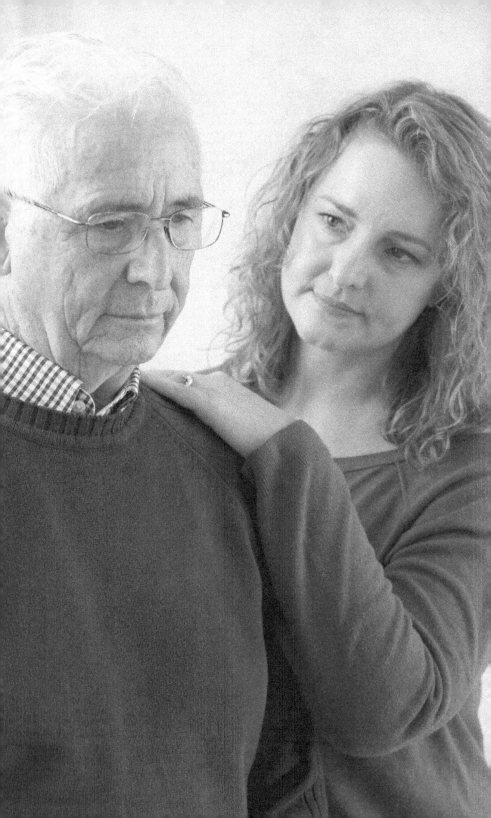

QUESTION #22

Is there research on the relationship between hearing loss and dementia?

Research conducted by Dr. Frank Lin and his team at Johns Hopkins Medical Center revealed age-related hearing loss is a major risk factor for dementia. People who experience hearing loss are 200-500% more likely to develop dementia than those with normal hearing.

Summary data of the relationship between hearing loss and increased risk of developing dementia.

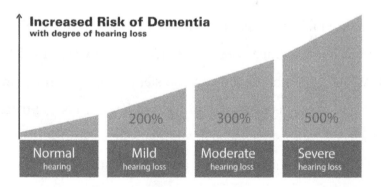

Dr. Lin commented on the issue, stating, "A lot of people ignore hearing loss because it's such a slow and insidious process as we age. Even if people feel they are not affected, we're showing that it may be a more serious problem."

The loss of receptor cells in the ear can be related to hearing damage, including a decrease in the number and quality of neural connections from the ear to the brain. The results usually impair memory, hearing, speech, and language.

Some serious factors associated with hearing loss and dementia include:

- Social Isolation
- Cerebral Atrophy
- Cognitive Overload

Social Isolation (The Impact of Withdrawal)

Most individuals with hearing loss naturally shy from social situations due to cumbersome surroundings. Many studies cite that people feel embarrassed or avoid starting conversations. In this retreat, it begins even in mild cases of hearing loss. In these instances of diminished social activity, physical exercise also suffers. All factors involved may lead to dementia.

"Blindness Separates You from Things, Deafness Separates You from People". ~~ Helen Keller

Cerebral Atrophy (AKA Brain Shrinkage)

The association of a shrinking brain, resulting from the loss of neurons, with dementia has been long documented. Even people with Mild Cognitive Impairment (MCI) show signs of cerebral atrophy. In recent years, scientific studies using advanced brain imaging techniques (including FMRI-Functional Magnetic Resonance Imaging) have demonstrated that hearing impairment is associated with accelerated brain atrophy, with advanced reductions in volume associated with the memory, hearing, speech, and language portions of the brain.

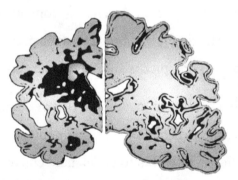

Brain With Hearing Loss   Brain With Normal Hearing

Schematic representing the potential cerebral atrophy in an individual with age-related hearing loss.

Cognitive Overload (Working Your Brain Too Hard in Order to Hear)

The term *cognitive overload* may appear harmless, but it can cause permanent damage to the person's brain function if left unchecked.

The person may even jokingly comment, "I need to put on my glasses so that I can hear you better."

While this might seem like a natural recourse, overall, this reliance on visual and lip-reading cues may take a toll on one's cognitive functioning.

When hearing is impaired, the strain of the brain continually attempting to decipher and comprehend the conversation is simply too much. Hearing loss places constant stress on the brain to fill in the missing pieces and follow the conversation.

High cognitive load is linked to a higher risk of dementia. Pupillometry measures mental effort using pupil size and can show how hard the brain works to understand conversations. Recent studies reveal that people who address their hearing loss have an easier time listening (lower cognitive load) and can remember up to 20% more of a conversation, even in noise.

QUESTION #23

Can my risk of developing dementia be reduced by treating hearing loss?

People suffering from hearing loss increase their risk of developing dementia. However, not all hope is lost. Hearing aids have been found to help reduce this risk. Additionally, interacting with friends and family, regular physical exercise, maintaining an active social life, and engaging in mentally stimulating activities can also help reduce the risk of developing dementia.

Treating Hearing Loss and the Impact on Cognitive Function

According to the Lancet Commission on Dementia Prevention, Intervention, and Care, " . . . people with hearing loss who received hearing aid treatment experienced lower rates of cognitive decline, similar to individuals without hearing loss."

The report also stated that those with hearing loss showed lower levels of cognitive decline compared to those without hearing aids. Consequently, treating hearing loss is essential for maintaining normal cognitive functioning and reducing the risk of acquiring dementia in later life. Furthermore, early acceptance of hearing aids can help improve communication, social engagement, and cognitive functioning while preventing further decline in cognitive health.

Studies showed that cognitive functions such as recall, working memory, selective attention, and processing speed significantly improved in individuals in their 50s and 60s after starting hearing loss treatment. After two weeks of treatment, scores on those tests were shown to be enhanced, with participants responding faster and more accurately to questions (Glick, 2019). In short, a minimal time commitment to treatment yielded substantial cognitive benefits.

Treating Hearing Loss and the Impact on Risk of Developing Dementia

Since 2011, multiple long-term studies have provided strong evidence that treating hearing loss may eliminate the increased risk of developing dementia. Dr. Lalwani at Columbia University noted treating hearing loss . . .

. . .may offer a simple yet important, way to prevent or slow the development of dementia by keeping adults with hearing loss engaged in conversation and communication.

Perhaps the most definitive report comes from the Lancet Commission, which presented a new life-course model documenting potentially modifiable risk factors for dementia. The Commission's report suggests hearing loss is the most effective modifiable risk factor in preventing dementia. Other modifiable factors include reducing depression, increasing physical activity, and reducing social isolation-- each positively impacted by treating hearing loss.

QUESTION #24

Can I expect to be more socially active and engaged once I start treating my hearing loss?

Yes, treating hearing loss will allow an individual to increase their social engagement. Studies have shown individuals with untreated hearing loss often suffer from isolation, depression, and falling. Another important factor to consider is that hearing impairment can lead to a decrease in earning potential or unemployment risks.

Treatment of hearing loss can also help maintain important relationships with close friends or loved ones. The ability to act on social cues perceived through better hearing in any conversation is the foundation for cultivating meaningful connections.

A person's involvement in social, physical, economic, spiritual, and civic affairs all demand quality hearing. Thus, we must rely on preserving the values of socialization and reliance on loved ones to ensure active aging.

Other tips for active aging include:

- Share a meal with family and friends 3–5 times per week.
- Commit to an aerobics or exercise class.
- Learn a new hobby each year.
- Learn or continue to play a musical instrument.
- Join a book or special interest club.
- Participate in classes at your local senior center.
- Volunteer at a local hospital, church, or shelter.
- Go back to school.
- Go back to work.

As you can now understand, the benefits of treating hearing loss are significant in maintaining an active social life, as it enables effective communication wherever you go.

Connecting the Dots Between Treating Hearing Loss and Improving Quality of Life

Individuals who choose to treat hearing loss can increase physical activity, reduce stress and anxiety, help lose weight, and ultimately live a healthier and more independent lifestyle.

Improving hearing, either naturally or by using hearing aids, can increase the clarity of speech, improve the ability to follow a conversation with background noise, improve socialization skills, and reduce the risk of depression.

Hearing aids may help prevent a fall in older adults. A small amount of hearing damage can remove large parts of the soundscape around people, which leads to a greater risk of falls in those with hearing problems left untreated.

The debilitating effects of tinnitus can be minimized by treating hearing loss, increasing concentration, improving communication, leading to better sleep, and relieving negative thoughts and emotions.

The treatment of hearing loss is essential for maintaining normal cognitive functioning and reducing the risk of acquiring dementia in later life.

The basic concept revealed in Optimizing Brain Power is the significance of managing hearing loss, caring for your brain, and how they are linked. I wish you luck and happiness as you embark on the journey of treating hearing loss, restoring clarity, and increasing independence, all while keeping a healthy and fit brain! We look forward to seeing you at **Prescott Hearing Center**.

FAQs

A Guide of Frequently Asked Questions

What might happen if I wait to treat my hearing loss?

Any amount of hearing loss can cause major problems for several reasons. Dementia is correlated with hearing loss, as with several other diseases, including diabetes, coronary disease, kidney disease, and increased risk of falling. Early treatment also improves the prognosis and expected outcomes.

Who are some famous people who've invested in treating their hearing loss?

The list is quite long! An abbreviated list includes presidents Reagan, Clinton, and George H.W. Bush, and other celebrities and famous athletes, including Huey Lewis, Lou Ferrigno, William Shatner, Pete Townshend, Whoopi Goldberg, Derrick Coleman, Congressman Jim Ryun, Phil Collins, and Brian Kerwin.

Will I be able to afford hearing treatment?

Yes. Not only are hearing loss treatment options more affordable than ever, but insurance, payment plans, flexible spending accounts, and various other financing options make this a moot point.

Will being fit with hearing aids be painful or obvious to others?

No, and no. Advances in the miniaturization of technology have helped develop the most lightweight, discrete, and sometimes completely invisible technology ever used to treat hearing loss.

Will I miss work or other social activities once I am fit with hearing aids?

The initial comprehensive evaluation and treatment procedures will take between one and two hours. Follow-up visits will only take between fifteen and thirty minutes. Patients walk out of the office after the first appointment and go about their lives; only now they can hear much better.

Is it such a big deal if I don't treat my hearing loss?

Yes. Too many people believe their hearing loss is "normal for their age." "There is no such thing as 'normal' or 'age-corrected' hearing loss." Hearing loss is a progressive degenerative disorder that will continue to negatively impact your life and cognition the longer it goes untreated.

What are some warning signs that I may have hearing loss?

Early symptoms of hearing loss include difficulty following conversation in background noise, experiencing tinnitus (ringing in the ears), having to turn up the T.V. louder than others need it, asking people to repeat often, finding yourself needing to read lips to hear better, difficulty understanding on the phone, and your family bugging you about getting help.

What kind of side-effects can result from NOT treating my hearing loss?

Untreated hearing loss is connected to increased risk of falls, depression, and dementia, as well as increased stress and reduced physical activity. Hearing loss is common in people with diabetes, coronary disease, kidney disease, and depression,

Why should I choose a specialist to treat my hearing loss?

Hearing loss is a major medical condition and is the third most common medical disorder impacting seniors. Unfortunately, loopholes in many state and federal laws allow traditional hearing aids to be sold online and in retail establishments, including some big-box discount stores. These traditional hearing aids are often older models and are only designed to amplify sound.

Hearing Healthcare Professionals design a plan to treat cognitive aspects of hearing loss and is considered the 'gold standard' by offering 'best practices' by audiologists and board-certified specialists in private practice clinics.

What is a Patient Care Coordinator?

During your initial consultations, you will usually be assigned a patient contact person—we call this person a Patient Care Coordinator in our office—with whom to schedule appointments, confer for rescheduling and, of course, help answer any questions you may have up to this point.

Why are follow-up visits important?

These are wonderful opportunities to ask questions, get further details from your specialist, or bring a family member to learn about your diagnosis and treatment plan.

Why is early treatment of hearing loss so important?

We recommend adults ages fifty and older have a comprehensive hearing evaluation. At fifty, if the patient has hearing loss, it is critical to start treatment early to avoid the devastating consequences of untreated hearing loss. Alternatively, if the patient has normal hearing, a baseline will be established and used for comparison at follow-up appointments.

What if I don't believe in early treatment of age-related hearing loss?

Unfortunately, for many patients, it takes nearly seven years to admit they have a hearing loss (or succumb to pressure from family members) and start treatment. By this time, the hearing loss will typically be moderate or beyond, and in some cases, treatment outcomes can be negatively impacted. To assure a positive prognosis and improved treatment outcomes, hearing loss must be caught early and treated to maintain positive connections to the brain. "Catch it early and treat it early!"

What is sensorineural hearing loss?

Sensorineural hearing loss (SNHL) is a hearing impairment that results from damage or dysfunction of the inner ear (cochlea) and/or the auditory nervous system. Age-related hearing loss is a form of sensorineural hearing loss.

What is conductive hearing loss?

Conductive hearing loss (CHL) is a hearing impairment that results from damage to, or dysfunction of, the outer ear (pinna and ear canal) and/or the middle ear (the eardrum or ossicles—

hammer, anvil, and stirrup). In some cases of CHL, medical or surgical intervention can help restore hearing function.

What is a processing disorder?

Hearing loss is often defined by the amount of lost volume that results from either an SNHL or a CHL. However, many patients, even those with normal hearing levels, can have a processing disorder that will limit their ability to understand and follow speech in background noise. The noise cancellation feature in prescriptive hearing aid technology provides significant benefits by reducing background noise and enhancing speech—even for those with normal hearing.

Should I bring a family member to my appointment(s)?

The answer is YES. Your hearing loss impacts not only you, but everybody around you. I have always encouraged every patient to bring a spouse or loved one to every appointment. The person can help the provider and the patient better understand the daily impact of hearing loss on everyone's life. It is also important to assess how your family member speaks. Are they 'soft talkers' or do they really mumble? Also, having another interested person understand the technical features of the technology can be beneficial for further support when you go home with your new devices.

87

What are the primary benefits of hearing aids?

- Binaural processing (two ears working together),
- Sound orientation (ability to detect the source of incoming sounds with increased accuracy)
- Enhanced clarity of voices (even soft speakers), automatic adaptation to the environment (no more pushing buttons and adjusting volume)
- Noise-cancellation filtering of background noise to enhance hearing conversation in noisy environments (hearing better in crowded rooms, restaurants, etc.)

In summary, recent reports find that hearing aids can significantly improve quality of life, reduce the risk of developing dementia, decrease the risk of falls, increase cognitive function, and reduce the negative effects of tinnitus. All these issues can be achieved by treating hearing loss with hearing aids.

How do I start treatment?

It's simple: request an appointment with **Prescott Hearing Center** by calling our office at (928) 237-2525 or visiting www.prescotthearing.com. We offer a free initial consultation to see if you are a suitable candidate for hearing loss treatment.

Epilogue

If you have questions, we hope that *Optimizing Brain Power* has provided answers.

So, there you have it! Twenty-four common questions that I get frequently asked about hearing loss and its effect on one's health. For your convenience, I have also included a handy FAQ section that summarizes most, if not all, of the questions we've just covered.

The fact is, no book can answer every question for each patient. People are unique, just like every patient with hearing loss. Therefore, **Prescott Hearing Center** provided this basic overview so you can be more confident in asking the right questions while visiting a hearing healthcare provider.

To take the next step, schedule your hearing evaluation and consultation with **Prescott Hearing Center**. Office number: (928) 237-2525.

About the Author

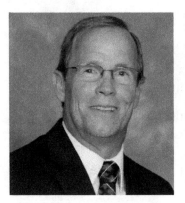 Doug Dunker is the founder and principal at **Prescott Hearing Center**. In 1999, he received a diploma in Hearing Instrument Sciences from Bates College in Tacoma, Washington. In 2004, he became board-certified in Hearing Instrument Sciences (BC-HIS), and in 2013, he received a certificate from the International Hearing Society for completion of the American Conference of Audioprosthology (ACA) course. He also holds a Bachelor of Business Administration from Globe University and an MBA from Minnesota School of Business.

Since Doug has tinnitus himself, he takes a special interest in providing tinnitus treatment options to his patients. By receiving a Tinnitus Care Provider certificate from the International Hearing Society, he can offer guidance and care to others who also suffer from tinnitus.

Doug is licensed to dispense hearing aids in Arizona and Utah and proudly offers educational seminars to the community relating to the negative effects of hearing loss and the benefits of available treatment options.

At **Prescott Hearing Center**, we focus on providing quality services and premium products from the most respected manufacturers in the industry. Our advanced testing, fitting, and verification equipment is guaranteed to provide the highest performance and satisfaction of any treatment solution.

Our commitment is to provide friendly advice and recommendations for hearing care solutions to assist clients throughout their hearing healthcare journey.

References

The Science Behind Everything
You Read in This Book

Optimizing Brain Power is the result of my 25 years in hearing health care. During this time, I have amassed information from my research, read scientific publications, in professional meetings, and directly interact with patients and their loved ones. Below is a list of references that helped me put together this book and present the information to you in a succinct manner. You can access these manuscripts on Google Scholar and/or PubMed.

- "Active Ageing: A Policy Framework." The Aging Male 5, no. 1 (2002), 1-37.
- Adult Cognition and Hearing Aids. U of Canterbury. Communication Disorders, 2015.
- Agmon, Maayan, Limor Lavie, and Michail Doumas. "The Association between Hearing Loss, Postural Control, and Mobility in Older Adults: A Systematic Review." Journal of the American Academy of Audiology 28, no. 6 (2017), 575-588.
- "Association of Hearing Impairment and Subsequent Driving Mobility in Older Adults." The Gerontologist 55, no. Suppl_2 (2015), 137-138.
- Bainbridge, Kathleen E., Howard J. Hoffman, and Catherine C. Cowie. "Diabetes and Hearing Impairment in the United States: Audiometric Evidence from the National Health and Nutrition Examination Survey, 1999 to 2004." Annals of Internal Medicine 149, no. 1 (2008), 1.
- Bassuk, Shari S., Thomas A. Glass, and Lisa F. Berkman. "Social Disengagement and Incident Cognitive Decline in Community-Dwelling Elderly Persons." Annals of Internal Medicine 131, no. 3 (1999), 165.
- Bernabei, Roberto, Ubaldo Bonuccelli, Stefania Maggi, Alessandra Marengoni, Alessandro Martini, Maurizio Memo, Sergio Pecorelli, Andrea P. Peracino, Nicola Quaranta, and Roberto Stella. "Hearing loss and cognitive decline in older adults: questions and answers." Aging Clinical and Experimental Research 26, no. 6 (2014), 567-573.
- Burns, Elizabeth R., Judy A. Stevens, and Robin Lee. "The direct costs of fatal and non-fatal falls among older adults — United States." Journal of Safety Research 58 (2016), 99-103.
- Cardin, Velia. "Effects of Aging and Adult-Onset Hearing Loss on Cortical Auditory Regions." Frontiers in Neuroscience 10 (2016).
- Cass, SP. "Alzheimer's Disease and Exercise: A Literature Review." Curr. Sports Med. Rep, February 16, 2017.
- Chen, David S., Dane J. Genther, Joshua Betz, and Frank R. Lin. "Association Between Hearing Impairment and Self-Reported

Difficulty in Physical Functioning." Journal of the American Geriatrics Society 62, no. 5 (2014), 850-856.

- Chia, Ee-Munn, Jie J. Wang, Elena Rochtchina, Robert R. Cumming, Philip Newall, and Paul Mitchell. "Hearing Impairment and Health-Related Quality of Life: The Blue Mountains Hearing Study." Ear and Hearing 28, no. 2 (2007), 187-195.

- Collins, John G. "Prevalence of Selected Chronic Conditions: United States, 1983- 85." PsycEXTRA Dataset (n.d.).

- Davidson, JGS. "Older Adults With a Combination of Vision and Hearing Impairment Experience Higher Rates of Cognitive Impairment, Functional Dependence, and Worse Outcomes Across a Set of Quality Indicators." Last modified August 1, 2017.

- De Leon, M. J., S. DeSanti, R. Zinkowski, P. D. Mehta, D. Pratico, S. Segal, C. Clark, D. Kerkman, J. DeBernardis, and J. Li. "MRI and CSF studies in the early diagnosis of Alzheimer's disease." Journal of Internal Medicine 256, no. 3 (2004), 205-223.

- Deal, Jennifer A., Josh Betz, Kristine Yaffe, Tamara Harris, Elizabeth Purchase Helzner, Suzanne Satterfield, Sheila Pratt, Nandini Govil, Eleanor M. Simonsick, and Frank R. Lin. "Hearing Impairment and Incident Dementia and Cognitive Decline in Older Adults: The Health ABC Study." The Journals of Gerontology Series A: Biological Sciences and Medical Sciences, 2016, glw069.

- "Dementia Prevention, Intervention, and Care." Lancet, July 19, 2017.

- Desjardins, Jamie L. "Analysis of Performance on Cognitive Test Measures Before, During, and After 6 Months of Hearing Aid Use: A Single-Subject Experimental Design." American Journal of Audiology 25, no. 2 (2016), 127.

- Ferreira, Lidiane M., Alberto N. Ramos, and Eveline P. Mendes. "Characterization of tinnitus in the elderly and its possible related disorders." Brazilian Journal of Otorhinolaryngology75, no. 2 (2009), 249-255.

- Genther, Dane J., Joshua Betz, Sheila Pratt, Kathryn R. Martin, Tamara B. Harris, Suzanne Satterfield, Douglas C. Bauer, Anne B. Newman, Eleanor M. Simonsick, and Frank R. Lin. "Association Between Hearing Impairment and Risk of Hospitalization in Older

Adults." Journal of the American Geriatrics Society 63, no. 6 (2015), 1146-1152.

- Gibrin, PC, AN Ramos Junior, and EP Mendes. "Prevalence of Tinnitus Complaints and Probable Association with Hearing Loss, Diabetes Mellitus and Hypertension in Elderly." Codas, 2013.
- Gispen, Fiona E., David S. Chen, Dane J. Genther, and Frank R. Lin. "Association Between Hearing Impairment and Lower Levels of Physical Activity in Older Adults." Journal of the American Geriatrics Society 62, no. 8 (2014), 1427-1433.
- Govender, SMS, CD Govender, and G. Matthews. "Cochlear Function in Patients with Chronic Kidney Disease." South African/Commun Disord, December 2013.
- Haan, Mary N. "Can Social Engagement Prevent Cognitive Decline in Old Age?" Annals of Internal Medicine 131, no. 3 (1999), 220.
- "Hearing Impairment and Frailty in English Community-Dwelling Older Adults: A 4-Year Follow-Up Study." The Gerontologist 56, no. Suppl_3 (2016), 319-319.
- "Hearing Loss and Cognitive Decline in Older Adults." JAMA Internal Medicine, February 25, 2013.
- "The Impact of Hearing Loss on Quality of Life in Older Adults." Gerontologist, October 2003.
- "The Impact of Hearing Loss on Quality of Life in Older Adults." Gerontologist, October 2003.
- "An Introduction to MarkeTrak IX: A New Baseline for the Hearing Aid Market." Hearing Review, May 15, 2015.
- Jacoby, R., and R. Levy. "CT Scanning and the Investigation of Dementia: A Review." J.R. Soc. Med, May 1980.
- Jamaldeen, Jishana, Aneesh Basheer, Akhil Sarma, and Ravichandran Kandasamy. "Prevalence and patterns of hearing loss among chronic kidney disease patients undergoing hemodialysis." Australasian Medical Journal, 2015, 41-46.
- Kamil, Rebecca J., Lingsheng Li, and Frank R. Lin. "Association between Hearing Impairment and Frailty in Older Adults." Journal of the American Geriatrics Society 62, no. 6 (2014), 1186-1188.
- Kelley, Amy S., Kathleen McGarry, Rebecca Gorges, and Jonathan S. Skinner. "The Burden of Health Care Costs for Patients With

Dementia in the Last 5 Years of Life." Annals of Internal Medicine 163, no. 10 (2015), 729.

- Kochkin, Sergei. "MarkeTrak VII." The Hearing Journal 60, no. 4 (2007), 24-51.
- Lambert, Justin, Rouzbeh Ghadry-Tavi, Kate Knuff, Marc Jutras, Jodi Siever, Paul Mick, Carolyn Roque, Gareth Jones, Jonathan Little, and Harry Miller. "Targeting functional fitness, hearing and health-related quality of life in older adults with hearing loss: Walk, Talk 'n' Listen, study protocol for a pilot randomized controlled trial." Trials 18, no. 1 (2017).
- Le Goff, Nicolas, Dorothea Wendt, Thomas Lunner, and Elaine Ng. "Opn Clinical Evidence. Oticon White Paper." 2016.
- Lin, F.R., L. Ferrucci, Y. An, J.O. Goh, Jimit Doshi, E.J. Metter, C. Davatzikos, M.A. Kraut, and S.M. Resnick. "Association of hearing impairment with brain volume changes in older adults." NeuroImage 90 (2014), 84-92.
- Lin, Frank R. "Hearing Loss Prevalence in the United States." Archives of Internal Medicine171, no. 20 (2011), 1851.
- Lin, Frank R. "Hearing Loss and Falls Among Older Adults in the United States." Archives of Internal Medicine 172, no. 4 (2012), 369.
- Lin, Frank R., E.J. Metter, Richard J. O'Brien, Susan M. Resnick, Alan B. Zonderman, and Luigi Ferrucci. "Hearing Loss and Incident Dementia." Archives of Neurology 68, no. 2 (2011).
- Martini, Alessandro, Alessandro Castiglione, Roberto Bovo, Antonino Vallesi, and Carlo Gabelli. "Aging, Cognitive Load, Dementia and Hearing Loss." Audiology and Neurotology 19, no. 1 (2014), 2-5.
- Meister, Hartmut, Stefan Schreitmüller, Magdalene Ortmann, Sebastian Rählmann, and Martin Walger. "Effects of Hearing Loss and Cognitive Load on Speech Recognition with Competing Talkers." Frontiers in Psychology 7 (2016).
- Melse-Boonstra, Alida, and Ian Mackenzie. "Iodine deficiency, thyroid function and hearing deficit: a review." Nutrition Research Reviews 26, no. 02 (2013), 110-117.

- Meyerhoff, William L. "The Thyroid and Audition." The Laryngoscope 86, no. 4 (1976), 483-489.
- Miyawaki, Christina E., E. D. Bouldin, G. S. Kumar, and L. C. McGuire. "Associations between physical activity and cognitive functioning among middle-aged and older adults." The Journal of Nutrition, Health & Aging 21, no. 6 (2016), 637-647.
- Mulrow, Cynthia D., Christine Aguilar, James E. Endicott, Ramon Velez, Michael R. Tuley, Walter S. Charlip, and Judith A. Hill. "Association Between Hearing Impairment and the Quality of Life of Elderly Individuals." Journal of the American Geriatrics Society 38, no. 1 (1990), 45-50.
- Oh, Esther, Frank Lin, and Sara Mamo. "Enhancing Communication in Adults with Dementia and Age-Related Hearing Loss." Seminars in Hearing 38, no. 02 (2017), 177-183.
- Palmer, Andrew D., Jason T. Newsom, and Karen S. Rook. "How does difficulty communicating affect the social relationships of older adults? An exploration using data from a national survey." Journal of Communication Disorders 62 (2016), 131-146.
- Popelka, Michael M., Karen J. Cruickshanks, Terry L. Wiley, Theodore S. Tweed, Barbara E. Klein, and Ronald Klein. "Low Prevalence of Hearing Aid Use Among Older Adults with Hearing Loss: The Epidemiology of Hearing Loss Study." Journal of the American Geriatrics Society 46, no. 9 (1998), 1075-1078.
- Qian, Z. J., Peter D. Chang, Gul Moonis, and Anil K. Lalwani. "A novel method of quantifying brain atrophy associated with age-related hearing loss." NeuroImage: Clinical 16 (2017), 205-209.
- Qian, Zhen J., Kapil Wattamwar, Francesco F. Caruana, Jenna Otter, Matthew J. Leskowitz, Barbara Siedlecki, Jaclyn B. Spitzer, and Anil K. Lalwani. "Hearing Aid Use is Associated with Better Mini-Mental State Exam Performance." The American Journal of Geriatric Psychiatry 24, no. 9 (2016), 694-702.
- Ryu, Nam-Gyu, Il J. Moon, Hayoung Byun, Sun H. Jin, Heesung Park, KyuSun Jang, and Yang-Sun Cho. "Clinical effectiveness of wireless CROS (contralateral routing of offside signals) hearing aids." European Archives of Oto-Rhino-Laryngology 272, no. 9 (2014), 2213-2219.

- Seimetz, Bruna, Adriane Teixeira, Leticia Rosito, Leticia Flores, Carlos Pappen, and Celso Dall'igna. "Pitch and Loudness Tinnitus in Individuals with Presbycusis." International Archives of Otorhinolaryngology 20, no. 04 (2016), 321-326.
- Sindhusake, Doungkamol, Paul Mitchell, Philip Newall, Maryanne Golding, Elena Rochtchina, and George Rubin. "Prevalence and characteristics of tinnitus in older adults: the Blue Mountains Hearing Study: Prevalencia y características del acúfeno en adultos mayores: el Estudio de Audición Blue Mountains." International Journal of Audiology 42, no. 5 (2003), 289-294.
- Snapp, Hillary A., FredD. Holt, Xuezhong Liu, and Suhrud M. Rajguru. "Comparison of Speech-in-Noise and Localization Benefits in Unilateral Hearing Loss Subjects Using Contralateral Routing of Signal Hearing Aids or Bone Anchored Implants." Otology & Neurotology 38, no. 1 (2017), 11-18.
- "Social Isolation in Community-Dwelling Seniors: An Evidence-Based Analysis." Health Quality Ontario, August 2008.
- Spulber, Gabriela, Eini Niskanen, Stuart MacDonald, Oded Smilovici, Kewei Chen, Eric M. Reiman, Anne M. Jauhiainen, Merja Hallikainen, Susanna Tervo, and Lars-Olof Wahlund. "Whole-brain atrophy rate predicts progression from MCI to Alzheimer's disease." Neurobiology of Aging 31, no. 9 (2010), 1601-1605.
- Su, Peijen, Chih-Chao Hsu, Hung-Ching Lin, Wei-Shin Huang, Tsung-Lin Yang, Wei-Ting Hsu, Cheng-Li Lin, Chung-Yi Hsu, Kuang-Hsi Chang, and Yi-Chao Hsu. "Age-related hearing loss and dementia: a 10-year national population-based study." European Archives of Oto-Rhino-Laryngology 274, no. 5 (2017), 2327-2334.
- Vignesh, S. S., V. Jaya, Anand Moses, and A. Muraleedharan. "Identifying Early Onset of Hearing Loss in Young Adults with Diabetes Mellitus Type 2 Using High Frequency Audiometry." Indian Journal of Otolaryngology and Head & Neck Surgery 67, no. 3 (2014), 234-237.
- Weinstein, Barbara E. Hearing Impairment and Social Isolation in the Elderly. Publisher not identified, 1980.

- Yates, J.A., L. Clare, and B. Woods. "You've Got a Friend in Me: Can Social Engagement Mediate the Relationship Between Mood and MCI?" Innovation in Aging 1, no. suppl_1 (2017), 1179-1179.
- Yates, Jennifer A., Linda Clare, and Robert T. Woods. "What is the Relationship between Health, Mood, and Mild Cognitive Impairment?" Journal of Alzheimer's Disease 55, no. 3 (2016), 1183-1193.
- Zheng, Yuqiu, Shengnuo Fan, Wang Liao, Wenli Fang, Songhua Xiao, and Jun Liu. "Hearing impairment and risk of Alzheimer's disease: a meta-analysis of prospective cohort studies." Neurological Sciences 38, no. 2 (2016), 233-239.

Printed in the USA
CPSIA information can be obtained
at www.ICGtesting.com
JSHW010050051023
49553JS00004B/16